THIS LOG BOOK BELONGS TO:

_____

_____

DATE	TIME	BLOOD PRESSURE		HEART RATE (PULSE)	NOTES
		SYSTOLIC (UPPER #)	DIASTOLIC (LOWER #)		

DATE	TIME	BLOOD PRESSURE		HEART RATE (PULSE)	NOTES
		SYSTOLIC (UPPER #)	DIASTOLIC (LOWER #)		

DATE	TIME	BLOOD PRESSURE		HEART RATE (PULSE)	NOTES
		SYSTOLIC (UPPER #)	DIASTOLIC (LOWER #)		

DATE	TIME	BLOOD PRESSURE		HEART RATE (PULSE)	NOTES
		SYSTOLIC (UPPER #)	DIASTOLIC (LOWER #)		

DATE	TIME	BLOOD PRESSURE		HEART RATE (PULSE)	NOTES
		SYSTOLIC (UPPER #)	DIASTOLIC (LOWER #)		

DATE	TIME	BLOOD PRESSURE		HEART RATE (PULSE)	NOTES
		SYSTOLIC (UPPER #)	DIASTOLIC (LOWER #)		

DATE	TIME	BLOOD PRESSURE		HEART RATE (PULSE)	NOTES
		SYSTOLIC (UPPER #)	DIASTOLIC (LOWER #)		

DATE	TIME	BLOOD PRESSURE		HEART RATE (PULSE)	NOTES
		SYSTOLIC (UPPER #)	DIASTOLIC (LOWER #)		

DATE	TIME	BLOOD PRESSURE		HEART RATE (PULSE)	NOTES
		SYSTOLIC (UPPER #)	DIASTOLIC (LOWER #)		

DATE	TIME	BLOOD PRESSURE		HEART RATE (PULSE)	NOTES
		SYSTOLIC (UPPER #)	DIASTOLIC (LOWER #)		

DATE	TIME	BLOOD PRESSURE		HEART RATE (PULSE)	NOTES
		SYSTOLIC (UPPER #)	DIASTOLIC (LOWER #)		

DATE	TIME	BLOOD PRESSURE		HEART RATE (PULSE)	NOTES
		SYSTOLIC (UPPER #)	DIASTOLIC (LOWER #)		

DATE	TIME	BLOOD PRESSURE		HEART RATE (PULSE)	NOTES
		SYSTOLIC (UPPER #)	DIASTOLIC (LOWER #)		

DATE	TIME	BLOOD PRESSURE		HEART RATE (PULSE)	NOTES
		SYSTOLIC (UPPER #)	DIASTOLIC (LOWER #)		

DATE	TIME	BLOOD PRESSURE		HEART RATE (PULSE)	NOTES
		SYSTOLIC (UPPER #)	DIASTOLIC (LOWER #)		

DATE	TIME	BLOOD PRESSURE		HEART RATE (PULSE)	NOTES
		SYSTOLIC (UPPER #)	DIASTOLIC (LOWER #)		

DATE	TIME	BLOOD PRESSURE		HEART RATE (PULSE)	NOTES
		SYSTOLIC (UPPER #)	DIASTOLIC (LOWER #)		

DATE	TIME	BLOOD PRESSURE		HEART RATE (PULSE)	NOTES
		SYSTOLIC (UPPER #)	DIASTOLIC (LOWER #)		

DATE	TIME	BLOOD PRESSURE		HEART RATE (PULSE)	NOTES
		SYSTOLIC (UPPER #)	DIASTOLIC (LOWER #)		

DATE	TIME	BLOOD PRESSURE		HEART RATE (PULSE)	NOTES
		SYSTOLIC (UPPER #)	DIASTOLIC (LOWER #)		

DATE	TIME	BLOOD PRESSURE		HEART RATE (PULSE)	NOTES
		SYSTOLIC (UPPER #)	DIASTOLIC (LOWER #)		

DATE	TIME	BLOOD PRESSURE		HEART RATE (PULSE)	NOTES
		SYSTOLIC (UPPER #)	DIASTOLIC (LOWER #)		

DATE	TIME	BLOOD PRESSURE		HEART RATE (PULSE)	NOTES
		SYSTOLIC (UPPER #)	DIASTOLIC (LOWER #)		

DATE	TIME	BLOOD PRESSURE		HEART RATE (PULSE)	NOTES
		SYSTOLIC (UPPER #)	DIASTOLIC (LOWER #)		

DATE	TIME	BLOOD PRESSURE		HEART RATE (PULSE)	NOTES
		SYSTOLIC (UPPER #)	DIASTOLIC (LOWER #)		

DATE	TIME	BLOOD PRESSURE		HEART RATE (PULSE)	NOTES
		SYSTOLIC (UPPER #)	DIASTOLIC (LOWER #)		

DATE	TIME	BLOOD PRESSURE		HEART RATE (PULSE)	NOTES
		SYSTOLIC (UPPER #)	DIASTOLIC (LOWER #)		

DATE	TIME	BLOOD PRESSURE		HEART RATE (PULSE)	NOTES
		SYSTOLIC (UPPER #)	DIASTOLIC (LOWER #)		

DATE	TIME	BLOOD PRESSURE		HEART RATE (PULSE)	NOTES
		SYSTOLIC (UPPER #)	DIASTOLIC (LOWER #)		

DATE	TIME	BLOOD PRESSURE		HEART RATE (PULSE)	NOTES
		SYSTOLIC (UPPER #)	DIASTOLIC (LOWER #)		

DATE	TIME	BLOOD PRESSURE		HEART RATE (PULSE)	NOTES
		SYSTOLIC (UPPER #)	DIASTOLIC (LOWER #)		

DATE	TIME	BLOOD PRESSURE		HEART RATE (PULSE)	NOTES
		SYSTOLIC (UPPER #)	DIASTOLIC (LOWER #)		

DATE	TIME	BLOOD PRESSURE		HEART RATE (PULSE)	NOTES
		SYSTOLIC (UPPER #)	DIASTOLIC (LOWER #)		

DATE	TIME	BLOOD PRESSURE		HEART RATE (PULSE)	NOTES
		SYSTOLIC (UPPER #)	DIASTOLIC (LOWER #)		

DATE	TIME	BLOOD PRESSURE		HEART RATE (PULSE)	NOTES
		SYSTOLIC (UPPER #)	DIASTOLIC (LOWER #)		

DATE	TIME	BLOOD PRESSURE		HEART RATE (PULSE)	NOTES
		SYSTOLIC (UPPER #)	DIASTOLIC (LOWER #)		

DATE	TIME	BLOOD PRESSURE		HEART RATE (PULSE)	NOTES
		SYSTOLIC (UPPER #)	DIASTOLIC (LOWER #)		

DATE	TIME	BLOOD PRESSURE		HEART RATE (PULSE)	NOTES
		SYSTOLIC (UPPER #)	DIASTOLIC (LOWER #)		

DATE	TIME	BLOOD PRESSURE		HEART RATE (PULSE)	NOTES
		SYSTOLIC (UPPER #)	DIASTOLIC (LOWER #)		

DATE	TIME	BLOOD PRESSURE		HEART RATE (PULSE)	NOTES
		SYSTOLIC (UPPER #)	DIASTOLIC (LOWER #)		

DATE	TIME	BLOOD PRESSURE		HEART RATE (PULSE)	NOTES
		SYSTOLIC (UPPER #)	DIASTOLIC (LOWER #)		

DATE	TIME	BLOOD PRESSURE		HEART RATE (PULSE)	NOTES
		SYSTOLIC (UPPER #)	DIASTOLIC (LOWER #)		

DATE	TIME	BLOOD PRESSURE		HEART RATE (PULSE)	NOTES
		SYSTOLIC (UPPER #)	DIASTOLIC (LOWER #)		

DATE	TIME	BLOOD PRESSURE		HEART RATE (PULSE)	NOTES
		SYSTOLIC (UPPER #)	DIASTOLIC (LOWER #)		

DATE	TIME	BLOOD PRESSURE		HEART RATE (PULSE)	NOTES
		SYSTOLIC (UPPER #)	DIASTOLIC (LOWER #)		

DATE	TIME	BLOOD PRESSURE		HEART RATE (PULSE)	NOTES
		SYSTOLIC (UPPER #)	DIASTOLIC (LOWER #)		

DATE	TIME	BLOOD PRESSURE		HEART RATE (PULSE)	NOTES
		SYSTOLIC (UPPER #)	DIASTOLIC (LOWER #)		

DATE	TIME	BLOOD PRESSURE		HEART RATE (PULSE)	NOTES
		SYSTOLIC (UPPER #)	DIASTOLIC (LOWER #)		

DATE	TIME	BLOOD PRESSURE		HEART RATE (PULSE)	NOTES
		SYSTOLIC (UPPER #)	DIASTOLIC (LOWER #)		

DATE	TIME	BLOOD PRESSURE		HEART RATE (PULSE)	NOTES
		SYSTOLIC (UPPER #)	DIASTOLIC (LOWER #)		

DATE	TIME	BLOOD PRESSURE		HEART RATE (PULSE)	NOTES
		SYSTOLIC (UPPER #)	DIASTOLIC (LOWER #)		

DATE	TIME	BLOOD PRESSURE		HEART RATE (PULSE)	NOTES
		SYSTOLIC (UPPER #)	DIASTOLIC (LOWER #)		

DATE	TIME	BLOOD PRESSURE		HEART RATE (PULSE)	NOTES
		SYSTOLIC (UPPER #)	DIASTOLIC (LOWER #)		

DATE	TIME	BLOOD PRESSURE		HEART RATE (PULSE)	NOTES
		SYSTOLIC (UPPER #)	DIASTOLIC (LOWER #)		

DATE	TIME	BLOOD PRESSURE		HEART RATE (PULSE)	NOTES
		SYSTOLIC (UPPER #)	DIASTOLIC (LOWER #)		

DATE	TIME	BLOOD PRESSURE		HEART RATE (PULSE)	NOTES
		SYSTOLIC (UPPER #)	DIASTOLIC (LOWER #)		

DATE	TIME	BLOOD PRESSURE		HEART RATE (PULSE)	NOTES
		SYSTOLIC (UPPER #)	DIASTOLIC (LOWER #)		

DATE	TIME	BLOOD PRESSURE		HEART RATE (PULSE)	NOTES
		SYSTOLIC (UPPER #)	DIASTOLIC (LOWER #)		

DATE	TIME	BLOOD PRESSURE		HEART RATE (PULSE)	NOTES
		SYSTOLIC (UPPER #)	DIASTOLIC (LOWER #)		

DATE	TIME	BLOOD PRESSURE		HEART RATE (PULSE)	NOTES
		SYSTOLIC (UPPER #)	DIASTOLIC (LOWER #)		

DATE	TIME	BLOOD PRESSURE		HEART RATE (PULSE)	NOTES
		SYSTOLIC (UPPER #)	DIASTOLIC (LOWER #)		

DATE	TIME	BLOOD PRESSURE		HEART RATE (PULSE)	NOTES
		SYSTOLIC (UPPER #)	DIASTOLIC (LOWER #)		

DATE	TIME	BLOOD PRESSURE		HEART RATE (PULSE)	NOTES
		SYSTOLIC (UPPER #)	DIASTOLIC (LOWER #)		

DATE	TIME	BLOOD PRESSURE		HEART RATE (PULSE)	NOTES
		SYSTOLIC (UPPER #)	DIASTOLIC (LOWER #)		

DATE	TIME	BLOOD PRESSURE		HEART RATE (PULSE)	NOTES
		SYSTOLIC (UPPER #)	DIASTOLIC (LOWER #)		

DATE	TIME	BLOOD PRESSURE		HEART RATE (PULSE)	NOTES
		SYSTOLIC (UPPER #)	DIASTOLIC (LOWER #)		

DATE	TIME	BLOOD PRESSURE		HEART RATE (PULSE)	NOTES
		SYSTOLIC (UPPER #)	DIASTOLIC (LOWER #)		

DATE	TIME	BLOOD PRESSURE		HEART RATE (PULSE)	NOTES
		SYSTOLIC (UPPER #)	DIASTOLIC (LOWER #)		

DATE	TIME	BLOOD PRESSURE		HEART RATE (PULSE)	NOTES
		SYSTOLIC (UPPER #)	DIASTOLIC (LOWER #)		

DATE	TIME	BLOOD PRESSURE		HEART RATE (PULSE)	NOTES
		SYSTOLIC (UPPER #)	DIASTOLIC (LOWER #)		

DATE	TIME	BLOOD PRESSURE		HEART RATE (PULSE)	NOTES
		SYSTOLIC (UPPER #)	DIASTOLIC (LOWER #)		

DATE	TIME	BLOOD PRESSURE		HEART RATE (PULSE)	NOTES
		SYSTOLIC (UPPER #)	DIASTOLIC (LOWER #)		

DATE	TIME	BLOOD PRESSURE		HEART RATE (PULSE)	NOTES
		SYSTOLIC (UPPER #)	DIASTOLIC (LOWER #)		

DATE	TIME	BLOOD PRESSURE		HEART RATE (PULSE)	NOTES
		SYSTOLIC (UPPER #)	DIASTOLIC (LOWER #)		

DATE	TIME	BLOOD PRESSURE		HEART RATE (PULSE)	NOTES
		SYSTOLIC (UPPER #)	DIASTOLIC (LOWER #)		

DATE	TIME	BLOOD PRESSURE		HEART RATE (PULSE)	NOTES
		SYSTOLIC (UPPER #)	DIASTOLIC (LOWER #)		

DATE	TIME	BLOOD PRESSURE		HEART RATE (PULSE)	NOTES
		SYSTOLIC (UPPER #)	DIASTOLIC (LOWER #)		

DATE	TIME	BLOOD PRESSURE		HEART RATE (PULSE)	NOTES
		SYSTOLIC (UPPER #)	DIASTOLIC (LOWER #)		

DATE	TIME	BLOOD PRESSURE		HEART RATE (PULSE)	NOTES
		SYSTOLIC (UPPER #)	DIASTOLIC (LOWER #)		

DATE	TIME	BLOOD PRESSURE		HEART RATE (PULSE)	NOTES
		SYSTOLIC (UPPER #)	DIASTOLIC (LOWER #)		

DATE	TIME	BLOOD PRESSURE		HEART RATE (PULSE)	NOTES
		SYSTOLIC (UPPER #)	DIASTOLIC (LOWER #)		

DATE	TIME	BLOOD PRESSURE		HEART RATE (PULSE)	NOTES
		SYSTOLIC (UPPER #)	DIASTOLIC (LOWER #)		

DATE	TIME	BLOOD PRESSURE		HEART RATE (PULSE)	NOTES
		SYSTOLIC (UPPER #)	DIASTOLIC (LOWER #)		

DATE	TIME	BLOOD PRESSURE		HEART RATE (PULSE)	NOTES
		SYSTOLIC (UPPER #)	DIASTOLIC (LOWER #)		

DATE	TIME	BLOOD PRESSURE		HEART RATE (PULSE)	NOTES
		SYSTOLIC (UPPER #)	DIASTOLIC (LOWER #)		

DATE	TIME	BLOOD PRESSURE		HEART RATE (PULSE)	NOTES
		SYSTOLIC (UPPER #)	DIASTOLIC (LOWER #)		

DATE	TIME	BLOOD PRESSURE		HEART RATE (PULSE)	NOTES
		SYSTOLIC (UPPER #)	DIASTOLIC (LOWER #)		

DATE	TIME	BLOOD PRESSURE		HEART RATE (PULSE)	NOTES
		SYSTOLIC (UPPER #)	DIASTOLIC (LOWER #)		

DATE	TIME	BLOOD PRESSURE		HEART RATE (PULSE)	NOTES
		SYSTOLIC (UPPER #)	DIASTOLIC (LOWER #)		

DATE	TIME	BLOOD PRESSURE		HEART RATE (PULSE)	NOTES
		SYSTOLIC (UPPER #)	DIASTOLIC (LOWER #)		

DATE	TIME	BLOOD PRESSURE		HEART RATE (PULSE)	NOTES
		SYSTOLIC (UPPER #)	DIASTOLIC (LOWER #)		

DATE	TIME	BLOOD PRESSURE		HEART RATE (PULSE)	NOTES
		SYSTOLIC (UPPER #)	DIASTOLIC (LOWER #)		

DATE	TIME	BLOOD PRESSURE		HEART RATE (PULSE)	NOTES
		SYSTOLIC (UPPER #)	DIASTOLIC (LOWER #)		

DATE	TIME	BLOOD PRESSURE		HEART RATE (PULSE)	NOTES
		SYSTOLIC (UPPER #)	DIASTOLIC (LOWER #)		

DATE	TIME	BLOOD PRESSURE		HEART RATE (PULSE)	NOTES
		SYSTOLIC (UPPER #)	DIASTOLIC (LOWER #)		

DATE	TIME	BLOOD PRESSURE		HEART RATE (PULSE)	NOTES
		SYSTOLIC (UPPER #)	DIASTOLIC (LOWER #)		

DATE	TIME	BLOOD PRESSURE		HEART RATE (PULSE)	NOTES
		SYSTOLIC (UPPER #)	DIASTOLIC (LOWER #)		

DATE	TIME	BLOOD PRESSURE		HEART RATE (PULSE)	NOTES
		SYSTOLIC (UPPER #)	DIASTOLIC (LOWER #)		

DATE	TIME	BLOOD PRESSURE		HEART RATE (PULSE)	NOTES
		SYSTOLIC (UPPER #)	DIASTOLIC (LOWER #)		

Made in the USA
Las Vegas, NV
27 December 2024

15473476R00056